BEYOND CANNABIS EXTRACTS

A Handbook to DIY Concentrates, Hash, and Original Methods for Marijuana Extract*s.*

Recipes for Bubble Hash, Dry Sieve, RSO (Rick Simpson Oil), Rosin tech and more.

Aaron Hammond

By Aaron Hammond

Version 1.1

Published by HMPL Publishing at KDP

Get to know yourpublisher and his work at

https://www.facebook.com/HMPL-publishing

A personal note from the writer

I have always been interested in cannabis and the medical benefits of marijuana so writing this book was a pleasure. As an aficionado in the cannabis world I came across hash and extracts years ago, as the quality of hash in Amsterdam was outstanding for that time this became my favourite product. Always eager to try new varieties and search for those excellent flavours, I've come across some of the best the cannabis industry has to offer.

In this book I will provide you with adequate and accurate knowledge about cannabis and traditional hash, as well as how this traditional hash is made and what the most common regions of production are around the world.

Ever since cannabis has been facing a lot of positive attention, the world of hash, extracts and concentrates has seen a massive boost, to where very high quality products became the market standard and people perfected the art of making them.

In this handbook I will explain the world of cannabis concentrates and we will go through the modern methods for extracts and concentrates and explain step by step how to it yourself!

I've always been somewhat of a MacGyver myself when it comes to production so I hope that these methods can spark some of that creativity in you if you don't have all the materials by hand.

With kind regards,

Aaron Hammond

Table of Contents

Bonus

Welcome to HMPL Publishing! Let's start right away with an exclusive bonus made available only for our inner circle. Get your free copy of 'The best DIY THC & CBD recipes to prepare at home' at eepurl.com\cxpVZf

Subscribing to our newsletter will guarantee you with the latest THC and CBD recipes, articles and some of our upcoming books for absolutely free. To make that even better we'll update you with the most recent information about Marijuana, medical breakthroughs and the various applications of cannabis. All you have to do is enter your email address to get instant access.

We don't like spam and understand you don't like spam either. We'll email you no more than 2 times per week. Here are some of the things you can expect as a subscriber to HMPL Publishing's newsletter:

To subscribe, go to eepurl.com\cxpVZf

A brief history of cannabis

Well we've all heard about it at least once in our lives, and recently with legalization across the United States it has become a hot topic. But that's not the place where we want to start off; we're going to go all the way back in history since cannabis has been known a long to humanity. Cannabis has always played an important role throughout time as medicine and later wrongfully accused as an illustrious drug ranking schedule I next to opioids.

It all started 12.000 years ago where cannabis plants are believed to have evolved on the steppes of Central Asia, specifically in the regions that are now Mongolia and southern Siberia, It is likely that these hemp and marijuana plants started to flourish on the nutrient-rich dump sites of prehistoric hunters and gatherers.

Over time archaeologists found burned cannabis seeds in kurgan burial mounds in Siberia dating back to 3000B.C. There were some of the tombs of noble people buried in the Xinjiang region of China that have had large amounts of the psychoactive marijuana buried with them. It was already used in China as an anaesthetic for surgery and stories even tell us that Chinese Emperor Shen Nung used cannabis around 2737 B.C.

Hailing from China about 2000 B.C. or earlier, there were coastal farmers that brought cannabis to Korea. Over time cannabis arrived to the South Asian subcontinent somewhere between 2000 B.C. and 1000 B.C., where at that time the region was invaded by the Aryans; a group that spoke an archaic Indo-European language. Over time as cannabis got more and more distributed around central Asia; the drug became widely used in India. They would celebrate cannabis in India as one of the five kingdoms of herbs which release us from anxiety according to one of the ancient Sanskrit Vedic poems whose name translate into; 'Science of Charms'.

How cannabis travelled from Asia to Europe

Between 2000 B.C. and 1400 B.C. cannabis arrived in the Middle East and there it was most likely used there by the Scythians, a nomadic Indo-European group. The Scythians are likely to be the ones that brought the herb into southeast Russia and Ukraine, as they have occupied both territories for years. Over time there have been Germanic tribes that brought cannabis into Germany, and marijuana went on from there to Britain during the 5th century with the Anglo-Saxon invasions taking most of the northern hemisphere in a couple of thousand years.

There have also been cannabis seeds that were found in the remains of old Viking ships dating back to the mid-ninth century where we can conclude that marijuana and hemp spread out over north-Europe as it first arrived in Germany and Russia.

Over the next following centuries, cannabis has travelled to various regions all over the world, traveling through Africa and spreading out over the course of years, where it reached South America in the 19th century and being carried north afterwards, eventually reaching North America.

How marijuana got into to the United States

After cannabis had travelled for a long time throughout the pre-modern and modern worlds, it finally arrived in the United States at the beginning of the 20th century. We discovered that cannabis crossed the border in the southwest United States when it came from Mexico, it was brought along with the immigrants fled their country during the Mexican Revolution of 1910-1911 seeking shelter in the United states.

There were many early prejudices against marijuana that have been thinly veiled racist fears of its smokers, often propagated by reactionary newspapers at that time. Mexicans were frequently blamed of smoking marijuana, accused of property crimes, engaging in murderous sprees and seducing children under the influence of marijuana. These claims were absolutely ludicrous but with lack of knowledge about the uses and effects of cannabis they were easily consumed by the masses giving the plant its illicit reputation.

The Americans laws have never recognized the difference between industrial hemp and the psychoactive marijuana. Utah was the first to outlaw cannabis in 1915. When Harry Aslinger became the first commissioner of the Federal Bureau of Narcotics in 1930, he made it his life duty to make cannabis illegal across all states. As time progressed and anti-marijuana regulations and laws were pushed all over the country; cannabis became illegal in 29 states by the end of 1931. A couple of years later in 1937, the Marijuana Tax Act came into place, putting cannabis under the regulation of the Drug Enforcement Agency, criminalizing possession of the plant throughout the country.

But things have changed over the course of time and as of January 2017, 29 states and the District of Columbia, starting with California in 1996, have legalized medical cannabis or effectively decriminalized it: Alaska, Arizona, Arkansas, California, Colorado, Connecticut, Delaware, Florida, Hawaii, Illinois, Maine, Massachusetts, Maryland, Michigan, Minnesota, Montana, Nevada, New Hampshire, New Jersey, New Mexico, New York, North Dakota, Ohio, Oregon, Pennsylvania, Rhode Island, Texas, Vermont, Washington; Maryland allows for reduced or no penalties if cannabis use has a medical basis. Despite the recent legalization of marijuana in Washington and Colorado, an employee can still be fired if they test positive on a drug test, despite having a valid doctor's recommendation.

California, Colorado, Connecticut, Arizona, New Mexico, Maine, Rhode Island, Montana, Michigan, Nevada and Oregon are currently the only states that have utilized dispensaries to sell medical cannabis; within the near future; Massachusetts, California and Nevada are planning to regulate selling recreational marijuana in dispensaries as they passed legalization in 2016. During 2008, California's medical cannabis industry took in about $2 billion and generated over $100 million in state sales taxes with an estimated 2,100 dispensaries, co-operatives, wellness clinics and taxi delivery services in the sector currently known by the abbreviation as "cannabusiness". As you might imagine this business is growing immensely with over $7 billion last year.

Now that we covered the part of history where you've learned how marijuana got its place in civilization; we can now move on to the next subject where we explain a part of the biology and chemistry of cannabis. The main course will be everything concerning cannabis extracts and concentrates as we will try to explain what they are in the most commonly known varieties and how they're made, the history behind them and how to do it yourself.

***

The biology of cannabis

Cannabis is the family name for a genus of a flowering plant that include three members know as cannabis sativa, cannabis sativa indica and the sub specie cannabis ruderalis commonly known as hemp.

As we learned from the history of cannabis, this plant is able to pretty much grow anywhere on this planet as long as it has sufficient light, humidity and nutrients. Cannabis has a long recorded use for hemp fiber, hemp oils, and medicinal purposes and as recreational drug. In its long history we learned that the early civilizations in Asia were the first to cultivate cannabis for medical use and many other purposes.

To start things off; Cannabis is an annual, flowering herb. Cannabis is dioecious which means that it is able to have male and female flowers on different plants of the same species. We won't get into detail on the subject of cannabis genders and reproduction as that is a subject for another time and another book but we do want to focus mainly on the two subspecies known as cannabis sativa and cannabis indica as these are used to make hash, concentrates and extract. Hemp or cannabis ruderalis isn't normally used because these plants don't contain a lot of THC, CBD and other compounds and industrial hemp is not bred to contain much of these psychoactive compounds.

So now that you know a little about the biology of cannabis we can get the most important part of the plants biology that's the vital ingredient of making hash, concentrates and extracts; the production of the resin that contains THC, CBD and other cannabinoids. Both cannabinoids and terpenes are manufactured in small resin glands present on the flowers and main fan leaves of late-stage cannabis plants called trichomes. This term is derived from the Greek word trikhōma, which means "growth of hair." Because both recreational and medical marijuana is bred and grown for their production of this psychoactive resin you can see the frostlike particles glistering with your bare eye but take a closer look and trichomes are nearly microscopic, mushroom-like protrusions from the surface of the buds, fan leaves, and in lower numbers the sticky glistering resin even appears on the stalk. While it is relatively complex to explain, trichomes are comprised primarily of a stalk and a head. It is within the head of the flower that the actual production of cannabinoids like THC and CBD occurs.

So the resin actually consists of three types of trichomes: Bulbous, capitate-sessile, and capitate-stalked. Bulbous trichomes are the smallest and you can barely see them without a microscope, as to where capitate-stalked, the largest variety of trichomes, are what most people notice when viewing their buds, either seen with the naked eye or under magnification. While more research is still necessary to reveal how these types are different from one another, it is commonly believed that these trichomes manufacture all types of cannabinoids and terpenes found in cannabis.

Trichomes are cannabinoid Factories

There are certain chemicals called vacuoles and plastids (which contain terpenes) that are manufactured in the stalks of the trichomes and travel up to the head of the gland. Once these chemicals arrive in the head, ultraviolet (UV) light will combine with them to help create cannabinoids. While this is a highly simplistic explanation, this helps to understand why plants that have received light of the proper wavelength, intensity, and duration are able to produce a greater volume of cannabinoids. When these cannabinoids happens to be THC, the euphoric and psychoactive potency of the plant increases.

However, it is necessary to mention that if you see a blanket of sugary trichomes on a particular sample of cannabis; it won't give you any certainty how strong the medical potential or psychoactive effects will be from that sample. While you can say that a great amount of resin glands on your flower is definitely a good sign, it doesn't necessarily mean that this glistering resin always contains a high percentage of THC, CBD, or other effective cannabinoids and terpenes.

To explain resin production from a biological perspective, it is commonly believed that trichomes evolved as a defence mechanism for cannabis plants, making it able to protect themselves from most threats in their natural environment, including insects and several animals. These trichomes make consumption of the plant less tasteful to hungry predators. Cannabis is also known to be able to inhibit some types of fungal growth and believed to protect the plant from forces of nature, helping it to survive against high wind and low humidity.

Resin: the source of hash, extracts and concentrates

We explained that trichomes are the microscopic factories in which cannabis produces cannabinoids and terpenes. These compounds derived from cannabis are the core material used in many types of cannabis extracts and concentrates. You might be familiar with kief, the powdery cousin of hash that basically contains a collection of decapitated trichome heads. The process of making hash is a similar type of extraction of trichomes where you intend to gather the cannabinoids and terpenes. Because most hash is pressed, the trichomes usually get crushed and the resin material co-mingles and begins to cure (at least on the outer sides of your product).

There are many ways to make hash but iceolator is one the more notorious types of hash, It's usually a very potent form of hash and made through the process of soaking cannabis leaves and flowers in bubble bags with ice water until the trichomes become frozen and brittle. So to extract the resin and get your iceolator you just have to shake it out in the bags so the trichomes detach and fall from the plant matter and are filtered and gathered by a fine micron sized screen at the bottom of your bubble bags. Shatter, BHO (butane hash oil), wax, and glass are simply different methods of collecting and processing the resin of the plant to produce a more potent medicine that involves less smoking and significantly higher percentages of coveted cannabinoids like THC and CBD.

When you extract and collect cannabis oil, you have the possibility to make cannabis oil infused edibles, capsules, or tinctures, these forms of medication can actually eliminate the need of smoking cannabis entirely while you're able to deliver a very potent dose of medicine in a discreet form factor.

So despite the celebration of the plant's green leaves and buds, you can say that it is actually the nearly invisible glistering crystalline resin of trichomes that provide all the medical or recreational value. So you must remember that it isn't the lovely green plant matter in their bowl or joint that is providing them with relief, but rather the sprinkling of resin glands on your buds which are the suspended compounds like THC and CBD.

We will go into specific methods to make hash, concentrates, extracts and everything about them later on in this book. We will explain the ins and outs about them, how to use them and make most of them yourself. So before we get into that; we are left with explaining the difference between cannabis sativa, indica and how those are crossbred to create hybrids and how each individual strain has its own known range of effects on the body and mind, resulting in a wide range of medicinal benefits.

***

The difference between indica and sativa strains

Indica

As you probably are familiar with the name by now; indica strains are known typically to grow short and wide. This growth pattern makes Indica plants very convenient for indoor growing. . The flowers or buds on an indica plant tend to grow shorter compared to sativa strains but usually very dense and compact and indica strains usually tend to produce heavier yields than sativa strains. There is a difference between indica and sativa when it comes to flavor and taste profiles; some differences in taste are very distinctive, some are more subtle and make it hard to define the difference by taste.

It is commonly believed that indica strains have originated in the Hindu Kush region near Afghanistan, where they have developed thick coats of resin as protection against the harsh climate and living conditions. Sativa plants tend to thrive in temperate and warmer areas closer to the equator.

Indica strains have great medical potential and they are very effective for overall pain relief and stress. Most patients benefit from indica strains to treat insomnia and increase their appetites. Indica buds are most commonly smoked by medical marijuana patients in the late evening or even right before bed due to how sleepy and tired you become when high from an indica strain of marijuana. The most popular Indica strains currently include several strains like Bubba Kush, Blueberry and Northern Lights.

Sativa

So as said before; sativa is the opposite from Indica plants, Sativa plants grow tall and thin, making them better suited for outdoor growing – especially since some strains can reach over 25 ft. in height. A Sativa high is known to be more energetic and uplifting.

Sativa-dominant marijuana strains tend to have a more grassy type odor to the buds providing an uplifting, energetic and "cerebral" high that is best suited for daytime smoking. A sativa high is one filled with creativity and energy as being high on sativa can spark new ideas and creations. It offers great medical potential to patients that suffer from ADHD and COPD as well as people that benefit from cannabis in general because sativa strains can help you get through the without the couch-lock from indica strains. There are many artists that like take advantage of the creative powers of cannabis sativa to create music, paintings and indulge in other forms of art. The most popular sativa strains include Sour Diesel and Purple Haze with reference to the great musician Jimi Hendrix.

Hybrids

Hybrid cannabis strains provide you the best of both worlds. Bred by experts in the business, these strains come from the best indica and sativa strains you can find to make even better and stronger ones. There are over 10.000 different strains of cannabis in general and hybrids maintain the best aspects from what both strains have to offer. Hybrids can be sativa or indica dominant and have the effects to match that offering great medical potential from both sides. Some of the most famous hybrid strains are Girl Scout Cookies, Blue Dream and OG Kush. Hybrid strains can vary between their sativa/indica ratio so effects can be different for every single plant. This principle goes for every strain whether they are indica, sativa or hybrid as for example; a strain might be generally known as a sativa but can have 70% indica phenol. We won't get into phenotypes and how that works as that is a subject for another book about growing cannabis.

***

A history of hash

The name hashish is derived from the Arabic word "حـ شـ يش"; which is the definition of grass and used as a word for cannabis. During the'60s a massive hashish production for international trade started coming from

Morocco and still is until present day. Cannabis plants are easily grown in Morocco and widely available especially around the Ketama region. A lot of farmers grow their product for export to Europe and you can legally buy imported morocco hashish in Amsterdam. Before the first hippies arrived from the Hippie Hashish Trail, you could only find small pieces hashish in Morocco. This product usually came from Lebanon back then because nobody was producing hashish in Morocco but business grew fast after people recognized the opportunity.

On the other side of the world and much closer to where cannabis and hemp originally came from there was the northern part of India that has a long social tradition in the production of hashish, known locally as Charas, which is believed to be the same plant resin that has been burned in the ceremonial boos room of Ancient Persia. You can find cannabis indica growing almost everywhere on the Indian sub-continent, and several strains such as Hindu Kush which we mentioned earlier have been cultivated for production of marijuana and hashish, especially in West Bengal, Rajasthan, the Hindu region and the Himalayas.

A long time ago in 1596, there was a Dutchman Jan Huyghen van Linschoten hailing from the Netherlands that wrote about his journeys and spent three pages on “bangue” (bhang) documenting the use of hashish in his time, especially around the Middle Eastern region where he mentioned Egyptian hashish? He wrote that bhang is likewise used in Turkey and Egypt, and is made in three varieties, carrying three different names. The first is known by the Egyptians and called Assis which means hashish in Arab, is the powder or kief derived from Hemp and cannabis, or the leaves, which is water made into paste or dough and they would eat five pieces, each piece as big as a Chestnut and sometimes larger; This is the way common people used hashish back in the day. As he wrote "because it is of a small price, and it is no wonder, that such virtue proceeded from the Hemp and Hemp excessively filled the head."

In the 1800s, hashish was used and embraced in some European literary circles. Most famously known, the Club des Hashischins was a Parisian club that dedicated themselves to the consumption of hashish and other drugs; the members included literary luminaries such as Théophile Gautier, Dr. Moreau 'de Tours, Victor Hugo, Alexandre Dumas, Charles Baudelaire and Honoré de Balzac. A French writer called Baudelaire later wrote the book Les paradis artificiels in 1860; in which he described the state of being under the influence of opium and hashish. At around the same time, American author Fitz Hugh Ludlow wrote the 1857 book The Hasheesh Eater about his youthful experiences, both positive and negative, with the drug.

So as you can see now; hashish has been part of cannabis culture for a very long time. Afghanistan leading is leading the world's hashish production right now distributing most of its product throughout the Middle East, Asia and Europe.

Original Moroccan hashish is very hard to come by in United States and if you can get your hands on some it usually comes at a hefty price. We will continue in the next chapters about the specifics of hash, extracts and concentrates and how to do it yourself!

***

Hash or Hashish

To start things off; we told you about the history of cannabis and hash in earlier chapters. Where hash has been produced, used and its role over the course of history. We mentioned that in several continents the product has a different name and is accordingly produced differently.

We'll dive deeper into that as we will explain the most common and traditional varieties of hash, where they come from and how they are made as well as explaining the modern forms of hash and methods of making them.

When it comes to testing quality if you got some hash of your own and you don't know much about it; here are the things that you should look for to decide if it's good quality hash.

Testing the quality of your Hash

Hashish produced in countries like Nepal, India and areas that surround the Himalayas has traditionally been made primarily by rubbing live marijuana flowers with hands or other implements as we will explain later on with our list of most common traditional hashish from around the world.

The aim is to get the soft and sticky resins to stick to a surface that can be taken somewhere to be processed. It is usually dark brown to black on the surface with a lighter colored interior. It can be adulterated with almost any type of oil including coconut and palm oils.

Middle East hashish from countries like Morocco, Turkey, and Lebanon is produced using the sieving process. The hashish is usually harder and drier than rubbed hashish. It can vary in color from yellow to red to brown.

If you break a piece open, you should see the very small granules of resin that make up hashish made by sieving. It can be adulterated with a variety of things like henna, tarmac, and can even include sand and tar extracts. But later on we will explain how burning the hash indicates its quality through consistency, ash and smoke.

You can usually tell rubbed and sieved hashish apart by the color and how pliable it is. Rubbed has a black or dark brown exterior and is more pliable when fresh. It also has a strong smell. Sieved hashish is golden yellow to red or light brown in color. It is drier (less pliable) than rubbed and the smell is more subtle. When you break a piece of dark to black hand –rubbed hash open it should show a greyish, green or brown like resin texture with a great smell to it if you have a good product. For sieved hash it should be light green to almost gold and the smell can be more subtle but applying heat to it with fire will definitely show the true colors or in this case quality when it melts or bubbles.

If you have the option of choosing; dry sift hash or bubble hash is almost always superior to hand-rubbed or traditionally pressed hah. Traditional hash that has been imported bears the risk that it has been mixed with other chemicals (usually oils) to increase its weight, but this decreases potency. Dealers would do this to increase their profit.

How pliable is good hand rubbed hashish? It should be harder at room temperature and become softer and more pliable after hand warming. Hold the piece in your hand for a few minutes. The higher the percentage of resin, the faster it will soften enough to be kneaded. Really hard hashish can be potent, but it is almost certainly far older and harsher.

How pliable is sieved hashish? Sieved hashish is usually a bit drier and harder than hand rubbed hashish, but should crumble fairly easily, in some cases turn in to powder.

The bubble test

By applying heat to your hash product the real quality will show, as great quality hash is made from only resin, just squeezing and kneading on body heat temperature it would already make it feel soft, oily, sticky and crumbly. In the best case it will full melt into oil when you apply heat using a lighter; meaning that it is the highest quality resin with a very high THC percentage(60% or more). As the quality goes down so does the ability to melt or bubble as that is an indicator of useless plant material or residue, or fillers if you got some bad quality stuff. From high to low quality it will melt, or bubble while partially turning in to oil while in bad cases in won't even show a single bubble or the hash won't even get soft. So the indicator of bubbles and oiliness is always a thing to look out for when testing the quality of your hash, but there are more indicators to decide what you got is good or not.

Smoke and ash

If you got some good full melt hash on your hands it should barely leave smoke as you would preferable dab it which means that this hash should just evaporate leaving very little to no residue behind. This is to indicate to highest quality possible because hash ranges from full melt to dark maybe even toxic smoke with very bad quality hash turning into some blackish ash. Indicators of good quality are light gray to almost white smoke and ash; the ash should be compact yet falling apart easily. With preferred bubbling oiliness in the process of burning; I never came across a piece of hash didn't bubble or showed some oiliness but turned straight up black to grayish white ash fire was applied. I don't think that just white ash without any of the other indicators is a good sign, same goes for oiliness and bubbles but the ash never turning white meaning that there is some material in the hash that shouldn't be there. Hash adulterated with oils and chemicals could show these signs as an indication of impurities. If you're making your own product you should always try to produce the highest quality product possible; because it is consumed by either smoking, vaping or using it for possible infusion and nobody should be willingly take in unwanted and maybe even very unhealthy materials.

***

Traditional types of hash

Below we will list the most common forms of traditional hash and their specifics.

Afghanistan

As we said earlier Afghanistan is currently one the biggest producers of traditional hash on earth right now with distribution to almost everywhere. Cannabis products from Afghanistan have a very long history of production dating back to 1926 where the Russian botanist Nikolai Vavilov documented some of the unique Afghani land strains that are still used in the production of hash

Traditional Afghan Hash

Cultivation: Hashish is produced practically everywhere in and around Afghanistan. The best kinds of hash originate from the Northern provinces between Hindu Kush and the Russian border in places like Balkh and Mazar-i-Sharif. As a tourist in Afghanistan it is nearly impossible to be allowed to see cannabis grow sites or the hash production.

Production: The plants which are used for hash production in Afghanistan are usually some short and bushy afghan landrace indica strain. In Afghanistan hashish is pressed by hand under addition of a small quantity of tea or water. The hash is worked on and kneaded until it becomes highly elastic and has a strong aromatic smell. In Afghanistan the product is stored in the form of Hash-Balls. Before being shipped, the hash is usually pressed in 100g slabs. Good quality slabs of Afghan hash are signed with the stamp of the producing family. Sometimes the hash slabs with those stamps are sold as Royal Afghan hash.

Color: Black on the outside, dark greenish or brown inside. Sometimes the hash can look kind of greyish on the inside; this is a sign of very high quality usually only seen in Afghan Temple Balls and Indian Charas

Smell: Spicy to very spicy.

Taste: Very spicy, it can be somewhat harsh on the throat. Afghan hash can induce lots of coughing in inexperienced users.

Consistency: Soft, usually can be kneaded very easily, sometimes hard and dry if it is really old, bad quality or both.

Effect: Almost narcotic because of the potency. It produces a very physical and stony high due to the indica origin of used strains.

Potency: weak to potent, sometimes very potent. It's easy to underestimate the potency of Afghani since the high takes about 5 minutes to reach its full potential. (6.5%-30% THC)

Availability: Quite rare, especially good qualities in United States. This hash is very common in Europe and along the way back to the Middle-East and Central-Asia.

Various: The softest Afghani isn't always the best; coconut or other oils are often added to soften the consistency in the originating country. There is also some Hash-Oil which is being produced from Afghani, the quality is usually excellent.

Afghan Temple Balls

Temple Ball Hash has become famous for its super sticky texture. This usually comes wrapped in cellophane or something similar to contain it. Otherwise this hash would stick to anything therefor being hard to remove and you'll lose some of that sticky goodness in the process. The oils within the Temple Ball Hash make it famous and providing its potency. Its origins lie in the regions of Afghanistan where tea houses were popular. As of these days you can find good black hash in pretty much every coffee shop in Amsterdam ranging from 5 to 12 euros for a gram but super-potent Temple Ball Hashish is still quite rare to come by.

Cultivation: The plants that are used usually the same as for regular afghan hashish.

Production: Making temple ball hash is done by rubbing dry marijuana flower tops between your hands. When the marijuana is cured and dried nicely, the resin will rub off quickly. This pile of resin containing loads of THC and cannabinoids is very sticky and can easily be molded into ball shapes. As they make this hash by hand you could see some skin cells in the pressed resin under a microscope.

Color: Black on the outside, should be grayish green on the inside

Smell: Spicy to very spicy.

Taste: sweet and tangy taste, this should be a very smooth smoke.

Consistency: Soft, can't be kneaded easily due to the hash being too sticky, oily and will stick to your fingertips.

Effect: Almost narcotic and dream inducing, treating insomnia and pain relief are its best medical benefits

Potency: very potent. Beware of underestimating the potency of Afghan Temple Balls (25 % - 60% THC in very rare cases even higher.)

Availability: Very Rare

India

Indian Charas Hash

Cultivation: Cannabis is cultivated nearly everywhere around the northern part of India.

Production: In India hash is produced by carefully rubbing the female buds between the hands. The resin is rolled in hash-balls, before shipment it's usually pressed in the slabs.

Color: Black on the outside, dark grayish/green inside.

Smell: Spicy to very spicy, usually a distinctive aroma.

Taste: Very spicy, should be a very smooth smoke if it's the real Charas.

Consistency: Very soft, can be kneaded easily like Afghani. Sometimes the hash can be quite powdery but it's always dense.

Effect: Very stony and physical high. Bears most of the effects of an indica but it can't be ruled out to induce a sativa high.

Potency: Potent to very potent. Like Afghan Temple Balls, Charas is almost always good smoke. (20-40% THC)

Availability: Very rare, almost never available outside the regions where it has been produced and most hash of this kind is imported by private travellers to India. Charas is usually sold locally as a 'finger', which is a sausage shaped piece of hash.

Lebanon

Red & Yellow Lebanese Hash

Cultivation: The most important grow-sites are located in the valley of Baalbek. The fields of cannabis are cultivated on a very large scale and many of them are using modern machinery. The production of this hash is very industrially oriented, traditional are usually not involved in the hash-business.

Production: The cannabis plants are left on the field until they are nearly dry. By the time they're dry you will see that the plants have turned into brown-reddish color because some chlorophyll is destroyed in the drying process by the UV-rays of the Sun. Finally the plants are brought in a barn to be dried completely.

Hashish is produced in the same way as in Morocco, basically the buds are carefully rubbed over a fine silk-cloth, and powder that you derive from the buds using this method can be pressed together. The size of the holes in your cloth; usually measured in microns decide the quality of your hash. We'll get into that with the method of dry sift hash as these methods are very similar to each other.

The kief or hash-powder is stored inside large plastic bags, so it can be kept for a long time without losing much potency.

When the winter starts, the pressing begins. Hash-Powder is filled in a linen or cotton bag and pressed under great pressure. On the surface of the Hashish the structure of the tissue that has been used to press this hash can be seen clearly. Usually this Hash is pressed in slabs of 100g, 200g or 1000g (1kg).

There is some Hash which is pressed by hand like in Afghanistan; unfortunately it's very rarely exported.

Color: There are two kinds of Lebanese-Hash: Yellow Lebanese, which is yellowish and Red Lebanese which is reddish-brown (very similar to standard Morocco in color). The Red-Lebanese is made from plants that have been cured and dried longer.

Smell: Spicy to very spicy, refreshing smell.

Taste: Very spicy, harsher than Turk or Morocco. Some Lebanese-Hash is harsher than Afghani, especially when smoked in a Bong. Lebanese hash is usually quite the acquired taste.

Consistency: The slabs of Lebanese hash are very thick (about 2-3cm) and not elastic or very sticky. However when you cut it, you can clearly see that it contains big quantities of resin and that it can be cut easily. Some kinds of Lebanese hash are more like Afghan hash and have the family stem on them. If you come across some exceptionally good Lebanese you should be able to re-press it by hand like Afghani due to its high resin-content.

Effect: The high is quite cerebral because it is probably more sativa dominant and the yellow variety of this hash produces a more cerebral high than the red kind (which has been cured better and contains more THC).

Potency: What you get from import is usually not very strong. The high resin content of the better varieties can be clearly seen and it can be re-pressed by hand. (1.0%-18% THC)

Availability: Quite rare, good qualities are very rare. However Lebanese is the third most common kind of Hash in Europe (after Morocco and Afghani). Unfortunately most of the Lebanese which is sold is quite old and dry, fresh and resinous Lebanese is very rare in the last years. Usually the price-range can be compared to that of Afghani.

Morocco

Traditional Moroccan Hash

Cultivation: Cannabis is usually grown on large sites in the northern regions of Morocco, especially in the province of Ketama. In 1992 farmers cultivated at least 30.000 acres of cannabis with growing numbers over time. This amount of cannabis accounts for about 15.000 tons of hashish which are exported to Europe; Coming in through Spain and distributed to France, Belgium, Holland, Germany, Switzerland and Italy.

Production: The cannabis flowers and for lower quality hash most of the remaining plant material is used. To make hash out of this; put this plant material on some fine silk-cloth in a bucket with the sides of the cloth tied over the bucket. Tie a large piece of plastic cover over the bucket covering it tightly so the plant material is between the plastic cover and the fine silk cloth. Now start drumming on the plastic cover with sticks but carefully enough not to damage the plastic cover but allowing the dried resin or kief to come off from the plant material and slip through the fine cloth into the bucket. The resulting powder can be pressed together. Lower Quality Moroccan Hash contains a lot of useless dried plant material that slipped through the cloth contributing to a very low THC percentage in the final product.

Color: Greenish to brown. Due to the relatively short growing season the plants retain a quite green color at harvest.

Smell: Lightly aromatic, not spicy.

Taste: Compared to other kinds of Hash the taste is usually very mild but it comes in many varieties such as blonde Maroc, caramello and since a couple of years there are strain specific varieties of Moroccan hash.

Consistency: can be quite variable, however generally the lower quality hash can be quite hard. Usually Maroc is sold in 0, 5 - 1,5cm thick slabs. General experience has taught me that you can't trust the name on any of the products as some rock hard pollen might be sold at coffeeshops in Amsterdam and some really good resinous oily soft pollen might be the same priced Maroc in another coffee shop.

Effect: Compared to other kinds of Hash it produces a quite cerebral and active high.

Potency: Regular cheap pollen is usually light to medium, only rarely potent. (0.9%-10% THC)

Availability: Moroccan is the most common kind of Hash on the European market; Morocco is sold under many names: varying from just Pollen of Polm, Hia, Super Maroc, Zero, Zero-Zero, King Hassan, Five Star Maroc, Warm Ears and probably many others.

Unfortunately these names aren't very useful, dealers sell everything which is slightly better than your average low quality Polm and put a fancy name on it, that's why I would recommend getting a strain specific piece of hash at a good coffee shop in Amsterdam because they usually got their own private supply of good quality hash from Morocco which is grown by demand.

I should add that botanically speaking the definition; Pollen is completely wrong. The hash is produced from female resin glands and not from male pollens which contain no THC.

Moroccan Caramello

Cultivation: The same as traditional hash but the difference lies in in the process of production

Production: This is generally produced the same way as traditional Maroc but the quality of the used plant material is much higher, generally using only flowers and top leaves to collect kief from instead of cutting to many corners with useless dried plant material as might be the case in cheap traditional Maroc. Keep in mind that there is no quality standard to this hash as names won't say much in an unregulated cannabusiness but the name caramello usually indicates higher quality Maroc.

Color: Dark greenish to brown

Smell: sweet and aromatic, usually a bit spicy with a slight scent of caramel and chocolate.

Taste: a good piece of caramello should taste the way it smells.

Consistency: should be on the soft side, with crumbling preferred over kneading. If it's old it can become quite dry but this usually doesn't take much away from the quality.

Effect: cerebral but relaxing stoned feeling.

Potency: Should be a lot better than your average cheap pollen. (15%-30% THC)

Availability: This is usually listed in many coffeeshops as the more expensive kind of hash and widely available around Amsterdam.

Moroccan Blonde Hash

Cultivation: The same as traditional hash but the difference lies in in the process of production

Production: This is generally produced the same way as traditional Maroc but the name indicates the color of the product which derives from fresher plant material thus giving its light green and usually more powdery consistency.

Color: Light green

Smell: sweet and aromatic, usually a bit spicy with a slight scent of tangy.

Taste: should be more tangy than sweet and slightly spicy but this depends on the quality and material used

Consistency: Usually bought hard pressed but it crumbles into powder if you try to break it. In very rare cases of high quality it should melt and bubble when burned.

Effect: cerebral and energetic sativa like high.

Potency: Should be a lot better than your average cheap pollen. (15%-30% THC)

Availability: Listed in many coffeeshops as the more expensive kind of hash and widely available around Amsterdam.

Moroccan strain specific Hash

Cultivation: Usually about the same as traditional Moroccan hash but the grow sites are a lot smaller as a single specific strain is used to produce this hash.

Production: This is generally produced the same way as traditional Maroc but the name of the final product indicates which strain has been used to produce the hash.

Color: all shades of green and brown to nearly black, depending on the strain and the process and duration of drying and curing the flowers.

Smell: If it's good quality you should definitely be able to smell the strain used to make this product.

Taste: depends on the strain used although there is usually some of that traditional Moroccan hash like spice to it.

Consistency: Usually bought pressed, but it should crumbles into sticky resin like powder if you try to break it or more soft and oily like some good quality Afghan but with the characteristics of traditional Maroc. Both crumble and oily are the indicators that you got should have some great quality product. This should definitely show some bubbles when burned and I have seen some amazing returns waxy concentrate if you Rosin Press a good piece of strain specific hash, indicating its high quality.

Effect: depending on the strain used.

Potency: a lot better than traditional varieties of Maroc. (25%-60% THC)

Availability: Listed in many coffeeshops as the most expensive kind of Moroccan hash and widely available around the better coffeeshops of Amsterdam.

Nepal

Traditional Nepalese Hash

Cultivation: There are small cannabis grow sites everywhere in the Highlands of Nepal.

Production: The resin is collected by carefully rubbing the buds between both hands. Later the collected resin is pressed to homogenous Hash-Balls (Like the Afghan Temple Balls and Charas). Before shipment these balls are pressed in slabs.

Color: Black on the outside, grey inside.

Smell: The aroma is very spicy, heavy and quite sweet. It is particularly potent if a piece of Hash is broken-up.

Taste: Highly aromatic and sweet, more so than Afghani but should be smooth on the throat like high quality Afghan

Consistency: Usually somewhat harder than Afghani but still soft enough to be kneaded at body temperature.

Effect: Very physical and indica stoney high

Potency: Potent to very potent. (25%-60% THC)

Availability: Very rare.

Most Nepal hash from Amsterdam is good quality Afghan sold under a different name. I've personally seen some of the real good Nepalese stuff and it is very rare to ever come across some and in the most cases if you don't get it locally in Nepal it has never that full certainty of knowing what you're actually dealing with; good Afghan might easily fool you.

Netherlands

Dutch hash

Cultivation: This hash is produced from Cannabis plants grown in the Netherlands. These plants are usually cultivated indoors but there are also small outdoor and greenhouse grow sites.

Production: The method to make this product varies with the producer of the hash. Most of the hashish is produced is through screening the kief like in Morocco, But some will always make some of that hand-rubbed hash produced using the Afghani method. However you should know that there it is only a small amount of the cannabis grown in the Netherlands that is processed in to hash.

Color: Usually quite green, however this varies with the strain of cannabis used and who produced it.

Smell: This is specific to the strain used, especially if it's made by screening: Dry sieve method which produces a very high quality hash.

Taste: Same as above.

Consistency: A lot of the Dutch hashish is not pressed as hard as imported products and usually beaks apart too easily. Often the hash is simply the female heads crushed and pressed under huge weights to form a solid lump which very easily powders up.

Effect: The kind of high depends from the strain of cannabis used, however usually the high is quite active and cerebral because the Dutch are known for their amazing sativa strains.

Potency: Potent to very potent, this stuff is usually better than any other kind of imported hash available to the average user. (Up to 90% THC) But this quality comes at a certain price.

Availability: rare outside the Netherlands and surrounding countries.

***

Modern methods of making hash

The methods of making hash haven't changed much recently; but the quality and efficacy has improved a lot, with legalization on the rise there is no need for cutting corners with low grade plant material and extremely potent and high quality products are available to a much larger audience of consumers. Now this doesn't take out the business of traditional hash with all its flaws as good quality imported hash will always have those unique taste characteristics unlike modern made dry sieve hash for example. But for real quality medicinal products you should definitely be looking at the modern way of making hash, which is transparent, can be legally produced and easily accessible in comparison to their mostly illegal traditional counterparts. Cultivators and extractors use the best flower now to make their product as competition in an open market demands for a high quality product. Which I personally think is the best thing that ever happened with legalization. In the following chapters of this book we talk about these methods and explain in easy steps how to do it yourself.

***

Bubblehash and Ice-o-lator

Ice-o-lator or Bubble hash is an extremely potent kind of hash. Bubblehash thanks its potency to its special method of production involving extraction and sieving through ice-water. Precise THC content is always a bit of a guess Unless you're able to have it tested, but Bubble hash is one of the more potent form of hash if you make it the right way.

Production

The secret behind bubble hash or iceolator is in the method of making it. Using iced water and agitation in special bubblebags, you are able to separate the resin from the buds, and from the icy water and then collect the resin. The trichomes and resin found on buds are oily so that means that they simply do not mix with water with makes the process actually pretty simple.

By putting about a 100 grams of good flower in iced water gives you 10 grams of very high-quality hash. It simply requires putting your weed in water, agitating it with an egg beater or cake mixer for 15-20 minutes and then using a filtration system of micron filtered bubblebags. These are a set of bags that come with different micron sizes for the filter part at the bottom of each bubble bag. Usually the bags are ranging with micron filters from 220μ up to 70μ with 70 microns being the finest filter able to sift through only the highest quality of crystals leaving you with a small amount of some very pure blonde resin. In the bags with ascending from 70 microns you will have left over residue of lower but still very high quality hash. We will explain this more thoroughly with dry sift hash as the method of extraction with bubble bags is fairly easy and the results are easily distinguished compared to dry sieve method.

Note: If you are using an electric mixing device, we recommend mixing in a separate bucket before pouring the mixture into your Bubble Bags and allowing it to settle.

The original Bubble Bag system which you can purchase online offers you eight layers of industrial grade micron filtration ranging from 220μ up to 70μ with 70 microns which will allow you to extract the perfect Bubble hash.

Supplies Needed:

-Good amount of great bud and top leaves

-Bubble Bag Kit

-Bucket

-Hand mixer or a spoon big enough to stir up your bucket

-Tea towel

-Pressing screen

Procedure

1. Line the bucket with your Bubble Bags, starting with the 25 micron bag and ending with the 220 micron bag.

2. Fill the bucket with enough cold water to cover the bottom of the Bubble Bags (about halfway full).

3. Add your dry or frozen plant trimmings.

4. Add enough ice to almost fill your bucket to the top.

5. Stir your mix for 15 to 20 minutes, adding ice if necessary to keep the water cold. A 50/50 mix of ice and water is ideal.

6. Pull out your Bubble Bags one by one, draining the leftover water in the bag into the bucket.

7. As you pull each Bubble Bag from the bucket, turn it inside out after it is finished draining to collect your herbal extract.

8. Gently press the excess moisture out of your bubble hash using your pressing screen and a dish towel.

***

Dry-sieve Hash

Dry sift or kief is the result of mechanically removing the resin glands from the plant by sieving them with screens of different sizes, without any kind of solvent.

So let's see how you can make the purest possible dry sift separation. We will use an ancient technique used in many of the traditional ways of hash making in which we sieve and re-sieve the resin glands with screens of different micron sizes. We can use either sieving screens or bags; if you want to use bubble bags without the ice and water to make dry sift hash it will be harder as you will have to screen very tense.

Most modern sieving systems on the market developed to separate resin glands, as the popular Pollinator, have a 150-160 micron mesh to separate the resin glands; which pass through the mesh from the plant material. But, according to the theory that a lot of plant residue isn't as small as the pure resin, there are lots of particles that also pass through the screen and that we don't want to be part of our hash. Therefore, you will need to use different screens with different micron sizes to continue separating the different qualities of particles of your raw resin. Normally, the best quality is where you find the higher proportion of trichome heads; larger than 70 microns and smaller than 120.

So, if you want the best possible quality results, filtering "downwards" with a 160 micron mesh is not enough. You should also perform a second sieve to get rid of those particles smaller than a certain size.

Supplies needed:

-Cured buds (amount depends on how much hash you want to make) 10 grams of good quality flower could potentially be 1 gram of quality sieve.

-Screen sieves in the sizes: 160, 70 and 45 microns

-oven plate (without anti stick! preferably glass, iron, ceramic.) or a large dish to catch the material derived from the sieving process.

-Grinder

Note: Always use a plate that's big enough to put the screens in as you don't want spill any of your product. Beforehand; you should make sure that your flower won't stick to the surface of the oven plate; No anti stick as you'll maybe have some kief that's a bit sticky but anti stick ruins everything!

Procedure:

1. Put the screens (ranging from 45 on the bottom to 160 on top) in the oven plate or large dish,

1. Break up and grind your flower

2. Put the flower straight from the grinder on to your 160 micron screen, and you can now either start sifting or grind more flower, repeating step 1 & 2

3. Start sifting your ground up material by spreading it around the screen and applying a little bit of tension but keep it gentle.

4. Sift al the material as good as possible until there are no particles that could be sieved through the 160 micron screen left.

5. Take off the 160 micron screen and put it carefully aside in a safe place; not spilling the material as you could use it to make cannabutter afterwards.

6. Repeat the process of sifting with resulting resin on your 70 micron screen to get your 70 micron dry sieve hash; as you sieve this thoroughly as explained in step 4.

7. Take off your 70 micron screen and carefully put that aside as this is your first quality dry sieve hash.

8. Repeat the steps of sifting with the resulting kief left on the 45 micron screen.

9. After sifting through the 45 micron screen you will have your second quality hash left on this screen; preferably you'd want to mix the first and the second

quality hash to get the best taste experience and effects, as the 45 microns contains more of the terpenes providing taste compared to THC trichomes in the 70 micron hash.

10. The small amount left on your plate or dish can be scraped together with something like a credit card and will be your third and highest quality dry sieve hash.

Drying and storing cannabis resin

The best dry sift hash is usually collected from buds cured for about 4-6 months (always, depending on phenotypes, drying and storage methods, etc.). We can cure our buds before making hash or just dry our buds, make the hash and cure the resin. Obviously, it is much more convenient curing and storing resin than plants.

Cured resin is pressed more easily than non-cured glands, and is also more potent and flavorful. The ideal curing temperature is 37°C, and we should open our jars every 2-3 days to renew the air inside them.

You can also store resin pressed. If you choose to do so, the resin will keep its organoleptic features much better, since only the surface will oxidize while the inside will degrade much more slowly. It is also advisable if you're planning to smoke the resin on a metal screen; otherwise, the resin will pass through it if you don't use several screens together. The ideal shape for minimum oxidation is a ball or sphere. Never press a piece of hash if you think there's moisture on the resin; cure it properly and then press it. Otherwise your hash can get spoiled in few days.

The best way to store our cured resin is inside an airtight container in the fridge, at low temperature and low humidity levels. If you want to store your hash for long periods with minimum degradation, and humidity; High temperatures and oxygen are the worst enemies so that's why the airtight container is definitely necessary

***

Scissor Hash and Finger Hash

Scissor or finger hash is the product of trimming wet cannabis plants. Cannabis flowers are very sticky due to the resin, especially when they still growing and wet. While handling and trimming plants, the resin stalks you know as trichomes get rubbed onto grower's hands, gloves and scissors. By rubbing the trichomes off, you essentially get yourself some high quality wet kief or often called live resin hash. The product is often a bit discolored compared to resin collected from dried and cured bud because it could contain some excess plant material, maybe some dirt and skin cells. This method of collecting hash could be compared to how traditional Charas and Nepalese hash is produced.

There is no need to go into explaining elaborate steps to produce this hash as this is probably the easiest way to do it, you'll need something like a small kitchen knife or a small scraping tool to collect the resin from your scissors used for trimming and some rubbing alcohol to clean up to scissors after you scraped off the live resin. Rubbing alcohol is needed because the resin will leave a thin but very sticky coating on the scissors and as this coating works the same as lipids, alcohol will help you dissolve the coating and get your scissors squeaky clean.

If you collect your hash by hand it can be quite the chore because it tends to be a very sticky process, so it will take you some time to roll your own had rubbed hash. You should try rolling a small ball or stick out of it that contains most of the resin collected on your hands and proceed to clean your hands afterwards with some good soap or rubbing alcohol; the latter being more effective and easier to clean with.

***

Cannabis extracts and concentrates

Cannabis concentrates and extracts have become ambiguous words in the cannabis industry recently. It could either refer to the wax you vaporize, the tincture used under your tongue, or the some of the many varieties of orally administered THC-free cannabis oil that has been changing attitudes toward cannabis everywhere in the past years. The future of cannabis is steering toward these potent concentrated forms, especially as the therapeutic potential of non-smoking methods is realized by the public.

Under the umbrella of cannabis concentrates falls any product procured through an extraction process. Extraction methods involving such as Butane, Alcohol and CO2 strip away the compounds from the cannabis plant, leaving behind a product with a very high concentration of cannabinoids packed in every drop. Some types of extracts have been tested as high as 90% in THC, while others are rich in non-psychoactive compounds like CBD and will deliver medical benefits to those who need CBD without inducing a high feeling whatsoever.

We have talked a lot about traditional hash varieties and methods to produce some very high quality hash yourself. Due to that high quality of dry sift and bubble hash you could definitely qualify them as extracts, especially if you would decide to purify them through a Rosin press. That would turn them into a more glass, was or shatter like substance, able to purify your hash from most of the plant matter left in your hash; purifying your extraction. But when it comes to traditional hash I wouldn't put the name concentrate or extract on it because if you got a piece of Moroccan hash that has been tested around 20% THC , you're talking about 80% residual plant matter and other possible contents in your product which don't exactly classify as an extract in my book. Technically speaking it is extracted but the quality is too low. Back in the day; when we're talking the 90's and earlier, there was only hash, very good hash and hash oil, the last one being a true extract in my opinion involving a solvent with a very high THC potency.

***

Traditional cannabis oil and methods

Traditional cannabis oils have been around for quite a while now and are made involving some kind of solvent; like Butane, Alcohol and CO2. The last one is basically the same method as Bubble hash; the bags are needed in the process but you take out water and use dry ice. We'll talk about that later; walking you through the steps of this method.

When we talk about traditional cannabis oils, there are two things that instantly come to mind being the well-known method for RSO or better known as Rick Simpson oil and the classic method of extracting cannabis oil with alcohol.

We'll talk first about measurements of THC and CBD contents in your extraction before we go into the methods of making cannabis oil. This is quite an important part of knowing what you're dealing with and finding the right dose of your cannabis extract.

***

Measuring THC in extracts and concentrates

The safest way of measuring how much milligrams of THC your cannabis extract contains is to have it lab tested but that is not always an available option. So here is a simple trick if you're in a situation where you need to measure it yourself. Please understand that this method of measure will not be the most accurate but it will help to indicate purity and dosage starting out with the plant material.

I would recommend using buds that are consumer-level grown medical cannabis if not for recreational purposes from certified dispensaries and farms. This means that that you're getting buds that are lab tested on their THC/CBD levels and you know how much % THC and CBD the cannabis contains in a gram.

Now provided that you have the choice between several different strains with the tested THC/CBD levels, you want to pick the strains that contain high CBD levels and low THC levels for CBD oil extraction. For people that are completely new to this; I have to explain that THC levels are independently different compared to CBD levels; 1-5% THC is considered to be a very low level of THC while 1-5% CBD is fairly high for a strain, so at the very high end of THC levels you should be looking at 15-25% THC per gram whereas the strains with a high CBD level are around 14-15% CBD. These amounts of compounds in cannabis are a key point in creating new strains of medical marijuana to grow buds with higher THC/CBD levels.

What you should be looking at ultimately for a good medical cannabis oil extract is a good CBD strain that has been tested with high levels of CBD ranging from 5-15% while THC remains at 5% and preferably lower. If you are growing marijuana yourself THC/CBD levels should be provided with the seeds of the strain when you're getting them from a professional cannabis seed company as they offer a great variety of high CBD/low THC level strains.

So you have the choice to pick the seeds that fit your need of medical marijuana. If you prefer a different balance of compounds, for example; you want high THC/very low CBD oil for daily use with the uplifting and energizing effects of THC the same rules of measurements are applied.

It all comes down to this: 1% of a single gram is 10 milligrams; so if you have a strain that contains 15% THC and 2% CBD we're looking at 150 milligrams of THC and 20 milligrams of CBD. This is the way to measure the buds you are using if they are lab-tested and THC/CBD levels are provided. If this is not the situation and you didn't grow it yourself or there is no way of ever testing it; you can't say anything about it.

You can speculate THC and CBD levels by the effect of using this cannabis. It's a general fact that high THC and very low to almost no CBD containing strains tend to give an uplifting, energizing, positive but could cause some anxiety. Whereas unknown strains or cannabis purchased illegally with slightly higher CBD levels (at the very rare maximum of 5% CBD per gram) usually gets you stoned. These strains will work relaxing, sedating, give you a couch-lock and work great against stress and anxiety.

It is almost completely impossible to ever encounter a pure CBD strain as recreational drug that is illegally sold on the streets as the effects are strictly medical and it won't get you high. These 5-15% CBD, 5% and lower THC strains will not make you feel high or stoned as CBD doesn't inhibit a psychoactive effect and it counters the psychoactive effect provided by the small amount of THC completely. The best way to get those strains is at your local dispensary or to grow them yourself.

Personally I cannot recommend ever buying marijuana illegally because it usually hasn't been tested; this cannabis bears the risks of containing pesticides or powders such as calcium, milk powder and other materials to improve the weight. There is a chance that glasslike glossy chemicals such as hairspray or simply glass powder has been used to make it appear like a densely THC covered nug or bud.

There is a risk that your illegally purchased and untested cannabis could be contaminated with PCP or other chemical drugs to improve effects and could be potentially very dangerous! This has in no way to do with the plant itself but it is one of the dark sides of drug business and a very urgent reason for legalization! Remind yourself that this part of the business is still illegal and usually doesn't have any concern for the user as there is money to be made.

Measuring the containments of cannabis oil itself.

Here is where it gets a little harder to get exact measuring on your own; if there is a possibility to get your oil lab tested, I urge you to do so as this method is not always very accurate. The larger the quantity of cannabis, the bigger your yield of cannabis oil will be and the easier it gets to measure the level of THC and CBD given that you have the right information at hand. So you will need to apply the same formula to calculate CBD and the contents are much easier weighted if they are larger.

So for example if you take a pound or 453 grams of lab-tested cannabis buds with 9,5% THC and 15,9% CBD you would technically speaking have 43,035 grams of THC (95mg of THC in a gram so 95 x 453 : 1000 =

43,035 grams of THC in pound of buds), The same principle applies to calculating the amount of CBD where you take the 159 mg of CBD in a gram, multiply that by the amount of cannabis so 453 grams and divide the outcome through a 1000 you should be looking at 72,027 grams of CBD in a pound of buds tested at 9,5% THC and 15,9% CBD. Now that we know this; you're looking at a potential 100% pure return in oil that should be 114,052 grams.

This would be extraction done to perfection and nearly impossible to achieve without the proper equipment, experience and knowledge.

As we will be using cheesecloth to strain the plant material and raw bud to makes this oil you will have plant residue left in your oil which will bring the concentration down, but I have seen, tested and used some very good homemade cannabis oils made by using this method that got lab-tested at a level of 70-95% of purity.

So you know what to look for now when you're making your own cannabis oil and want to measure the amounts of THC and CBD in your cannabis oil. But you want it to be exact. For example: You have tested your product so you're looking at 85% pure with 50% CBD and 35% THC in 100 grams of medical cannabis oil.

That means that you have about 15 grams of plant residue in your oil but the oil itself is very potent and of very high quality. If you know your math and if you're able to use the metric system this is will be very easy to calculate given that you are provided with the right information concerning the cannabis that you're using.

How to make Cannabis oil

Before you start anything you should read this: *This is a message from the writer urgent to everyone considering using this method to extract their own cannabis oil. As you are working with alcohol as a solvent it is of the utmost importance that you are aware of your surroundings concerning open fires, stoves smoking and other situations that could mean potential harm and risk of catching fire!*

This is an easy alcohol cannabis oil extraction method similar to the CBD extraction method in our book about CBD & Hemp-oil.

This process will yield you about two to four grams of extremely potent, medicinal-grade CBD oil that is suitable for ingestion. After you have a few practice runs, the entire process for small-batch edible oil production should take you about an hour, including around thirty minutes of cooking time. Grain alcohol is the solvent that is least likely to leave you impurities or residue in the final product.

Supplies Needed:

-One ounce of dried, ground-up bud material or two to three ounces of ground, dried trim/shake

-One gallon of solvent (Grain alcohol or other high-proof alcohol; **never use rubbing alcohol as there are chemicals in there to make this not suitable for human consumption and could potentially be very dangerous to your health!**)

-Medium-sized mixing bowl (Glass is best, or ceramic)

-Strainer (A cheesecloth/stainless steel kitchen sieve combo, or muslin bags, grain-steeping bags or even clean stockings/nylons)

-Catchment container

-Double boiler or au-Bain Marie

-Kitchen utensils (Large wooden spoon, silicon spatula, plastic syringe for dosage and dispensing of oil, funnel)

Your preparation area

-Heat Source: An electric stove in your kitchen would work well. It is more dangerous to use a gas stove (if that's what you have) since a gas stove uses an open flame - you must use extra caution with a gas stove as the flame can ignite your solvent - keep anything containing alcohol at least 3 feet away from the flame of a gas stove at all times. A portable electric burner or a large tea warmer also work well.

-Fire Extinguisher: you should already have one near your stove, but double-check to make sure it's there and not expired

-Ventilation: your preparation space should be a large open area with excellent ventilation. Open any windows and have at least one fan moving the air around. Turn on the fan above the stove if it's available. Solvent fumes in the air can catch fire, so the best thing you can do to protect yourself during this process is to ensure there is good ventilation in your preparation space.

Procedure

1. Get organized – Prepare your space, arrange your necessary equipment, find a level work area and make sure that it is clean and set up before starting

2. Place the ground-up Cannabis material into the mixing bowl, making sure to leave some space for the solvent. Find a larger bowl before proceeding further, if necessary.

3. Completely cover the plant material with the alcohol, adding about an extra inch of solvent above the top level of plant matter.

4. using the wooden spoon, agitate the Cannabis material within the solvent for about three minutes. This enables the resin glands to dissolve into the solvent. Make sure that the plant matter is thoroughly saturated and has had a chance to expel its resin content.

5. Place straining bag or sieve into the catchment container. Pour the dark green liquid from the mixing bowl into the bag or sieve; allow the liquid to be filtered completely and pour into the container. Gently massage the bag in order to squeeze out as much liquid as possible.

Note: At this point, you have the possibility to repeat the previous four steps in order to extract as much resin as possible into the solvent. This second wash should remove most of the remaining resin.

6.Pour the strained liquid into the double boiler or in the cooking pots(Au-Bain Marie; placing a smaller cooking pot in a bigger one, allowing to put water in the bottom pot to prevent the top pot from overheating or cooking to quickly). Fill the bottom of the double boiler or the bottom pot with an appropriate amount of water. If your alcohol-resin solution does not all fit in the top of the double boiler or cooking pot, you can keep refilling the pot as you boil down the CBD oil, eventually processing all of the rinse liquid.

7. Place the double boiler on high heat until the liquid begins to bubble, which is actually the alcohol evaporating. When it reaches the bubbling stage, turn off the burner – the residual heat contained in the water bath will continue heating the mixture, allowing the alcohol to evaporate.

8. If the mixture stops bubbling, it may be necessary to turn the heat back on, once or twice more. The evaporation step usually takes between fifteen and twenty-five minutes to complete.

Note: The mixture should continue bubbling throughout the evaporation process. As the alcohol level decreases, so will the amount of bubbles. It helps to occasionally mix the solution with the silicon spatula, scraping the sides of the pan as you mix.

***

Rick Simpson Oil

The Story of Rick Simpson

After Rick Simpson suffered from a serious head injury in 1997, Rick Simpson sought relief from his medical condition through the use of medicinal hemp oil. When Rick discovered that the oil with its high concentration of THC)cured cancers and other illnesses, he tried to share it with as many people as he could free of charge and start curing and controlling literally hundreds of people's illnesses.

Now we have gone a long way in legalization and use of cannabis ever since 1997, but the method of Rick Simpson oil is still relevant upon today for people who like their medicine this way so we will walk you through the steps of production. This method is similar to extracting cannabis oil with alcohol.

Method of making RSO (Rick Simpson Oil)

Before you start anything you should read this: *This is a message from the writer urgent to everyone considering using this method to extract their own cannabis oil. As you are working with alcohol as a solvent it is of the utmost importance that you are aware of your surroundings concerning open fires, stoves* *smoking and other situations that could mean potential harm and risk of catching fire!*

Supplies Needed

-One ounce of dried, ground-up bud material or two to three ounces of ground, dried trim/shake, Pick the strain that best fits your medical needs!

-One gallon of solvent (Grain alcohol or other high-proof alcohol**; never use rubbing alcohol as there are chemicals in there to make this not suitable for human consumption and could potentially be very dangerous to your health!**)

-Medium-sized mixing bowl (Glass is best, or ceramic)

-Strainer (A cheesecloth/stainless steel kitchen sieve combo, or muslin bags, grain-steeping bags or even clean stockings/nylons)

-Catchment container

-Double boiler or au-Bain Marie

-Kitchen utensils (Large wooden spoon, silicon spatula, plastic syringe for dosage and dispensing of oil, funnel)

Your preparation area

-Heat Source: An electric stove in your kitchen would work well. It is more dangerous to use a gas stove (if that's what you have) since a gas stove uses an open flame - you must use extra caution with a gas stove as the flame can ignite your solvent - keep anything containing alcohol at least 3 feet away from the flame of a gas stove at all times. A portable electric burner or a large tea warmer also work well.

-Fire Extinguisher: you should already have one near your stove, but double-check to make sure it's there and not expired

-Ventilation: your preparation space should be a large open area with excellent ventilation. Open any windows and have at least one fan moving the air around. Turn on the fan above the stove if it's available. Solvent fumes in the air can catch fire, so the best thing you can do to protect yourself during this process is to ensure there is good ventilation in your preparation space.

Procedure:

1. Gather supplies

Note: *Preparation is key! Make sure you have all the proper supplies ready BEFORE you get started. Make sure you have your double-boiler, your extra flat surface 3+ feet away from the stove, you cannabis (ground up), your bowl and a bottle of your chosen solvent.*

1. Place the ground-up Cannabis material into the mixing bowl, making sure to leave some space for the solvent. Find a larger bowl before proceeding further, if necessary.

2. Completely cover the plant material with the alcohol, adding about an extra inch of solvent above the top level of plant matter.

3. Use the wooden spoon and start to agitate the Cannabis material within the solvent for about three minutes. This will enable the resin glands to dissolve into the alcohol. Make sure that the plant matter is thoroughly saturated and has had a chance to expel its resin content.

4. Place straining bag or sieve into the catchment container. Pour the dark green liquid from the mixing bowl into the bag or sieve; allow the liquid to be filtered completely and pour into the container. Gently massage the bag in order to squeeze out as much liquid as possible.

Note: At this point, you have the possibility to repeat the previous four steps in order to extract as much resin as possible into the solvent. This second wash should remove most of the remaining resin.

5.Pour the strained liquid into the double boiler or in the cooking pots (Au-Bain Marie; placing a smaller cooking pot in a bigger one, allowing to put water in the bottom pot to prevent the top pot from overheating or cooking to quickly).

Fill the bottom of the double boiler or the bottom pot with an appropriate amount of water. If your alcohol-resin solution does not all fit in the top of the double boiler or cooking pot, you can keep refilling the pot as you boil down the CBD oil, eventually processing all of the rinse liquid.

6. Place the double boiler on high heat until the liquid begins to bubble, which is actually the alcohol evaporating. When it reaches the bubbling stage, turn off the burner – the residual heat contained in the water bath will continue heating the mixture, allowing the alcohol to evaporate.

7. If the mixture stops bubbling, it may be necessary to turn the heat back on, once or twice more. The evaporation step usually takes between fifteen and twenty-five minutes to complete.

Note: The mixture should continue bubbling throughout the evaporation process. As the alcohol level decreases, so will the amount of bubbles. It helps to occasionally mix the solution with the silicon spatula, scraping the sides of the pan as you mix.

If the liquid has stopped bubbling but is still runny, you may turn the heat back on low for a moment until it starts bubbling again. You should keep the heat just around the boiling point of alcohol.

Heat is not as important at this point. Even if this mixture cools down to room temperature which can be unlikely even in a cold room, the alcohol will all eventually evaporate away as long as you continue to stir.

8. You are done when the mixture stops boiling and takes on its consistency

While the oil is relatively soft now, once it cools down it will become thicker, almost like putty. You should work quick and steady to place this mixture into a plastic syringe, which will make it easy to store and dispense your medicine. Remember, this is a lot of medicine, and the starting dose is half the size of a grain of rice.

9. Use a plastic syringe to draw up the oil - this will allow you to easily create individual portions in the future

Quick Tip: Mix the warm cannabis oil with coconut or olive oil if you need to make less potent doses, or if you plan to use this topically on your skin.

For edible doses, you need to use plastic applicators or syringes with no needles. These are often used to dispense medicine for children, and can be found at the drug store or grocery store.

Use the plunger of the syringe to slowly draw up the warm cannabis oil. The first few syringes will be easy to fill, but as you have less and less liquid remaining in the pan, it will become harder. That's totally normal; just take your time and do your best.

If there is some amount of cannabis oil left which you cannot fit in a syringe, you can put the remaining oil in any sort of small closed container, and you will be able to use a toothpick to get tiny rice-sized pieces for individual portions after it cools.

The semi-runny oil will become much thicker after it cools - if the oil becomes too thick to push out of the syringe, simply run hot water over the syringe to soften the cannabis oil.

Store the cannabis oil in a cool, dark place such as a cabinet.

***

BHO's and the difference between shatter, glass, wax and budder

Shatter, wax, honeycomb, oil, crumble, sap, budder, pull-and-snap…these are some of the used nicknames that cannabis extracts have earned through their rising popularity, prevalence, and diversification. If you've heard any of those words anywhere before, they were likely used to describe BHO also known as butane hash oil, CO2 oil, or similar hydrocarbon extracts. This list of descriptive subcategories might lead you to believe that we are talking about some stark differences between each one, but the division between glass-like shatter and crumbly wax is more superficial than you would expect.

So we are talking different varieties of the similar substances derived through different methods; the most common method that has been related to these varieties called wax, shatter, glass and budder is BHO. Recent advancements in extraction technology have enabled the use of other solvent and over time a new method called Rosin developed as a method of solvent-less extraction. The end product derived through those methods is a highly potent oil of varying consistencies most popularly used for vaporization and dabbing.

Shatter, glass, wax and budder

Shatter, with its flawless amber glass transparency, has a reputation for being the purest and cleanest type of extract. But translucence isn't necessarily the way to tell signs of quality; the consistency and texture of oil comes down to different factors entirely.

The reason this shatter comes out perfectly clear has to do with the molecules which, if left undisturbed, form a glass-like appearance. Heat, moisture, and high terpene contents can also affect the texture, turning oils into a runnier substance that resembles sap; hence the commonly used nickname "sap". Cannabis oils that have the consistency that falls somewhere between glassy shatter and viscous sap are often referred to as "pull-and-snap."

The term wax refers to the softer, opaque oils in your concentrate that have lost their transparency after extraction. Unlike those of transparent oils, the molecules of cannabis wax have crystallized as a result of agitation. Light can't travel through those irregular molecular densities, and that refraction leaves us with solid, non-transparent oil.

Just as transparent oils span the spectrum between shatter and sap, wax can also take on different consistencies based on heat, moisture, and the texture of the oil. There are runny oils with more moisture that tend to form gooey waxes often called “budder,” while the harder ones are likely to take on a soft, more brittle texture known as “crumble” or “honeycomb.” The term “wax” can be used to describe all of these softer, solid textures.

How to make BHO

First, here are some very important bullet points you need to know first about what we can expect.

Equipment: you’ll need an extraction tube; these are available in different sizes according to the amount of material you want to use. Good quality butane preferably from the same shop as you’re getting your extraction tube from as not every other commercially sold can of butane is usable for cannabis extraction due to other chemicals that might be in this butane.

Yield: from frosty some good trim, you should be able to get at least 10% yield. That means that if you start with 100grams of product, you should get at least 10grams of shatter. From good bud you can yield up to 22-23% yield, but usually the results on flower is around 16-20% but that depends on the quality. With some less frosty strains, yields will be around 12-15%.

Material: If material is bad, end product will be bad. Plain and simple. You can’t take brick weed and expect it to make good shatter. However, you are able to get a great BHO from simple frosty trim if it's dried and cured properly. The frostier the material that you're using, the more yield you will get from it.

Safety: What you might have heard about the dangers of BHO is true! There is a lot that could go wrong, with the worst thing possible: igniting the butane fumes. Let's say that you're producing some BHO on your back porch and it starts to get dark. You flip on the light switch. If there is any kind of spark, those highly flammable fumes will ignite, explode, you'll be up dead and your house is wrecked. When you try to make BHO yourself, literally tape down the light switches so you or someone else can't accidentally turn on the light. Be sure to wear safety goggles. Butane will spatter out at some point, especially when you are still learning your equipment and finding the correct adapter from your butane can to the tube.

Supplies Needed

–10-oz can of butane per 1-oz of marijuana

– Extraction tube

– Medium Pyrex dish

– Large Pyrex dish

– Electric heating pad

– Razor blade scraper

– Concentrate container

– A purging system (optional)

Procedure:

1. Extract the marijuana. First of all, fill your extraction tube with the strain you have chosen to extract. Make sure to prevent any air pockets from forming and make sure the material you are using is extremely dry. Fill the tube, pack it down, and then repeat until your tube is full and air-free.

For less plant material, use a smaller tube.

2. Fasten the screen (or a mesh coffee filter) to the bottom of the tube. Hold it over the medium Pyrex dish, then get your butane and put the nozzle right over the top hole in the tube. Allow the butane to flow into the tube, and then wait for up to a minute until the liquid begins to drip into the Pyrex dish. Use as many butane cans as necessary. Allow the drip to continue for several minutes. The liquid that you collect in your Pyrex dish should appear gold in color.

3. Once you have completed the extraction process, you will need to evaporate the liquid so that the harmful butane can be removed. Get the large Pyrex dish and put the medium one inside of it. Then, put hot water in the outer, larger dish. This will cause the butane to begin to evaporate, which should take between fifteen and twenty minutes. Replace the hot water as needed to keep it hot. For your safety, be sure there is plenty of ventilation during this process.

4. Purge it. Purging is the process to complete the removal of the butane honey/hash oil. Using a purging system is the best way to do it, but many money-conscious people prefer to use an electric heating pad instead. Simply set it to high heat, and then place the medium Pyrex dish on it for an hour or more. Watch it carefully. This is finished once the oil stops bubbling.

Honey oil that has begun to become hazy or cloudy in appearance looks that way because of trapped butane. Purge it again to get rid of all the butane. One simple way of checking if there is any butane left in it is to touch it with a flame — if it catches, there is still butane that needs to be removed.

5. Store the oil. Use the razor blade scraper to get all of the oil out of the dish, and then put it all into a concentrate container. As long as it remains in an airtight container that remains dark and cool, BHO can last a long time. If improperly stored, you can expect the substance to become dry, tasteless, and less potent.

***

CO2 cannabis extraction

CO2 extraction is a method of extraction very similar to making Bubble hash with main and only difference that it takes using water out of the process by using dry ice.

Make sure you follow a few simple dry ice precautions while making your cold CO2 hash.

-Don't touch the dry ice without your gloves! You wouldn't want to get any freezer burns.

-Don't eat the dry ice.

-Don't place it in any airtight containers because you'll make them explode. Store it in a thick Styrofoam cooler to slow down the sublimation process.

-Make sure you work with dry ice in well-ventilated areas to avoid inhaling more carbon dioxide than you should.

-Safely dispose of any leftover dry ice by allowing it to warm up and transform back into harmless CO2 gas.

Supplies Needed:

-Good amount of great bud and top leaves

-Heat resistant gloves for handling the dry ice; you don't want to end up with freezer burns!

-Bubble Bag Kit in 220, 160, 120 and 70 microns.

-5 Gallon Bucket

- A putty knife, paint scraper or just a laminated card to collect the kief hash.

- A large clean mirror or piece of Plexiglas.

-About 3 pounds of dry ice

Procedure:

1. Safety first, put your gloves on.

2. Grind your cannabis up and drop it in your 5-gallon bucket.

3. Cover it in dry ice.

4. Fit your 70 micron bubble bag over the opening of the bucket and shake the contents around for about 4 minutes to freeze the trichome resin off of the cannabis.

6. Lift the bucket up, turn it upside down over your clean mirror or Plexiglas and start shaking out as much cold powdery resin through the micro-mesh bag as you can until you can't shake anymore out.

7. Use your scraper or card to smoothly scoop up the kief hash from your surface area into your mason jar.

8. Repeat the previous steps with the size-160 and 220 bubble hash bags in order to collect three different grades of pure, solvent-free, homemade CO2 hash which you can smoke, vape, dab or infuse into edibles!

***

Rosin tech method for extraction

Rosin Tech is by far the easiest method to extract your cannabis flower or any of your traditional hash and kief. It is a simple and affordable way to produce a quality product within seconds. This simple technique will separate the resin from the plant material by using heat and pressure. The resulting yields from this method are much similar to other extraction techniques, ranging between 10-15% with flower and much more with good quality hash like dry sift, bubble hash and kief.

Use the right tools

You can make rosin using most ordinary household hair straighteners or larger heat press systems such as t-shirt presses. Producing rosin press extracts requires a temperature between 240 and 330 degrees Fahrenheit on your ceramic plate. You will also need a heat source on both sides of the press. Any device that fits those criteria should work. You can purchase a hair straightener capable of making rosin for less than $20 for personal use. This is highly recommended for those planning on running up to a half ounce. Any more than that and you should look to invest in a heat press. This will run you several hundred dollars. The size of the ceramic plate on smaller devices matters less than you may think.

Small buds work the best if you're pressing cannabis flower

Think about it this way: using smaller nugs to press create more surface space overall. More surface space gives the resin a greater opportunity to reach parchment; the alternative being the oil will re-adhere to the starting material during the press. The good stuff collects in a ring around the starting material. Anything else is temporarily unobtainable unless you resort to running your chips over and over again. Doing this is not recommended. You will lose valuable terpenes each time you do this, so take the time to break your starting material down to 1/2 inch to 1/3 inch bits. You may spend more time pressing, but the end result of your extraction will be worthwhile.

Listen while you press

This may sound strange, but the sizzle coming from your press is a great way to gauge when sublimation is occurring; sublimation is the point at which the oils change from a liquid to a gaseous state and then begins to look for something non polar to adhere to. Most of the time, this will only takes about 5-7 second to hear this sizzle. After you hear it, let the pressure off a second or two later and remove the parchment from the heat source.

Temperature means everything!

Here is rough estimation that should help you with temperature.

Lower temperatures; 200's F, 90 -135 Celsius means more flavor, less yield, end material is more stable (shatter)

Higher temperatures; 300's F, 135 -185 Celsius means less flavor, more yield, end material is less stable and has a sap like consistency.

Do not go higher, this can be dangerous!

Use a screen to clean your extract

Get yourself a 25 Micron screen, because these are wonderful for processing kief and lower quality hash with. You can also use 90 micron tea filters to process flower with. Doing so will help keep all of the plant matter and particulates out of your end material. If you find that little pistils and other contaminants keep ending up in your flower rosin, use a dabber tool to remove them from the parchment before you collect. This should help!

Heat resistant Gloves

Heat resistant gloves cost less than 10 dollars and will ensure that you don't burn yourself. Practice safety always!

The difference between strains

Your flavour and yield begin with your starting material. If the flower has poor resin, you will produce poor hash oil. Garbage material in means garbage results out. Remember this if you find you aren't achieving adequate yields. Also, certain strains are known for producing better resin than others.

Before you collect it

After you press your starting material, let your parchment stabilize in the freezer for about 10 seconds. This helps with samples that lean towards the sappy side. Cooling it off will make it much more easier to collect your extract onto your dabber tool.

Use a ball point dabber tool to collect.

Ball point dabbers help you roll the tool over the paper. This ensures that you cover the most real estate. Sometimes, you might not be able to detect the rosin with your naked eye. However, rest assured that you are collecting material, even if you may not see it.

Supplies needed

- Any good amount of bud or quality hash

- Hair straightener with temperature control

- Non-stick parchment paper

- Collecting device such as a dabber tool, razor blade, etc.

- 25u micron screen

Procedure

1. Prepare your processing material by breaking it down to 0.2 - 0.5 inch increments. Cut 10-20 pieces of parchment paper in 4" x 8" strips. Preheat the flat iron to 200F/93 Celsius – 340F/171 Celsius.

2. Take one of the small increments that you prepared and wrap it in the center of the 25u micron screen. Place the screen with the product on a piece of parchment paper and then fold the paper over, leaving the product in the center of your parchment paper. Place the parchment paper on the flat iron and apply pressure for 3-5 seconds directly on the product.

3: Remove the pressure from the flat iron and take off the parchment paper, unfold the parchment paper. The starting product will be surrounded by the rosin, remove the product being careful to leave all of the rosin behind. Take your collecting device and scrape the parchment paper to collect the entire finished product.

***

Free Bonus

Subscribing to our newsletter will guarantee you with the latest THC and CBD recipes, articles and some of our upcoming books for absolutely free. To make that even better we'll update you with the most recent information about Marijuana, medical breakthroughs and the various applications of cannabis. All you have to do is enter your email address to get instant access.

We don't like spam and understand you don't like spam either. We'll email you no more than 2 times per week. Here are some of the things you can expect as a subscriber to HMPL Publishing's newsletter:

To subscribe, go to eepurl.com\cxpVZf

Thank you

Finally, if you enjoyed this book, then I'd like to ask you for a small favour. Would you be kind enough to leave an honest review for this book on Amazon? It'd be greatly appreciated by both the future reader and me!

You can find the book on Amazon.

Thank you and good luck!

www.ingramcontent.com/pod-product-compliance
Lightning Source LLC
Chambersburg PA
CBHW051813170526
45167CB00005B/1992
* 9 7 8 1 5 4 3 0 9 1 0 1 4 *